# The Paleo Diet for Rapid Weight Loss

## Loss Up To 30 LBS. in 30 Days

by FlatBelly Queens

Published in Great Britain by:

FlatBelly Queens
345 Old Street
London
EC1V 9LE

© Copyright 2016 – Flatbelly Queens

ISBN-13: {978-1533302182}
ISBN-10: {1533302189}

# Table of Contents

# Introduction:

It's an epidemic in this country: people are overweight, tired, and eat poorly. The American diet is full of carbohydrates, sugars, and processed foods, causing us to gain weight, feel malnourished, and too tired to do anything with our lives.

If you picked up this book, you are looking for a change. You are looking for a way to eat healthier and feel better. You also want to lose weight. You understand that the current Western diet just isn't working for you. Well, this book has the answer you seek.

Eat like a caveman! People refer to the paleo diet as

the caveman diet because it is based on how humans ate over 10,000 years ago, before the advent of agriculture. At that time, people ate what was available to them through hunting and foraging, which means meat, fruits, vegetables, and nuts. Dairy foods, carbohydrates, and anything processed were not available to them.

Eating like a caveman has many benefits, the biggest of which is that you will be healthier and will lose weight. It is our diet that causes us to carry so much extra weight, and by eating only healthy, unprocessed foods that our body was created to eat, you will lose weight! You will have more energy and feel better. It may take a little dedication to give up foods you are used to, but the results are more than worth it. Imagine being at a healthy weight for your body, having the energy to do all the activities you dream of, and feeling lean and mean, like the caveman of old.

You can lose weight. You can eat healthy. You can take control of your life. By eating the paleo diet, you will have all these things.

# Chapter 1: Benefits of Paleo

If you aren't sold yet on the benefits of the paleo diet, here are six benefits that the paleo diet has shown people.

## Weight Loss

The paleo diet is low carb, and eating too many carbs is the primary reason many people are overweight.

Carbohydrates do not fill you like meat does, and the energy released into your body is used quickly. So, shortly after you eat, you are hungry again. However, when you eat healthy, high protein foods that burn energy slowly, you feel fuller longer, eat less, and naturally lose weight. This is one of the big selling points of the paleo diet, and one of the best reasons to follow it. It helps you naturally lose weight without feeling starved or deprived!

## Better Intestinal Health

A diet high in processed foods, chemicals, and other junk can lead to stomach and intestinal issues, and can also cause what is called leaky gut, where foods in the intestines spill out to other parts of the body. But, eating a paleo diet prevents this from happening. The food stays in your intestinal tract, allowing you to get the nutrients from your food without adverse effects of the food itself. You'll also feel less bloating and intestinal discomfort.

## You'll Get Your Vitamins and Minerals

In the Western diet most of us eat today, we aren't getting enough of the vitamins and minerals our bodies need to run efficiently and effectively. However, because the paleo diet requires you to eat many fruits and vegetables, you will get more of the nutrients that your body needs to thrive. The paleo diet encourages a rainbow of colors in vegetables and fruits, which help ensure that you will get the vital nutrients most people miss on the current Western diet.

## Reduces Allergens from Your Diet

The paleo diet reduces allergens that are part of the current Western diet. Many people have issues digesting grains or dairy, and eating them can cause many health issues. People are so used to feeling the effects of these allergens, they may not even realize that they have food sensitivities. They just accept that this is how they are supposed to feel. The paleo diet removes these foods from your diet. If you are no longer suffering from food allergies, you'll automatically begin to feel better.

## Reduces Inflammation

Foods rich in omega-3 fatty acids have been shown to reduce the risk of inflammation in the body. Because the paleo diet is high in these omega-3 fatty acids, you will experience a reduction in inflammation. This can relieve many illnesses, such as rheumatoid arthritis, bronchitis, or even sinusitis. It can even help you reduce the severity of asthma due to its anti-inflammatory aspects. Plus, it has been shown that cardiovascular disease can be caused by

8

the inflammation of the arteries, so the paleo diet can even help prevent heart attacks and plaque build-up on your arteries!

## More Energy

Because you will be eating healthy, unprocessed, whole foods, you will naturally have more energy than eating a highly processed, grain-filled diet. You will eat food that burns slowly in your body, releasing energy over time, rather than the high followed by the crash of a diet high in carbs and sugars. You will have energy stores to get you through the entire day!

As you can see, the paleo diet can help with a variety of issues, make you feel better, and help you lose weight. You'll have more energy and be able to get through the day without artificial stimulants, such as caffeine or energy drinks. Plus, when you lose weight, one of the best benefits of the paleo diet, you will naturally have more energy and feel great!

# Chapter 2: Paleo Diet FAQs

## Is the paleo diet a scam?

The premise of the paleo diet is that before humans discovered agriculture about 10,000 years ago, they ate a very different diet. Humans, for 140,000 years only ate what they could hunt or forage, which meant meat, fish, fruits, vegetables, and nuts. Grains weren't even thought about as a food source. The paleo diet follows this plan. It worked for our ancestors for a very long time, and it is the most natural way to eat. This is how the human body was designed to eat, and getting back to it is the healthiest way to go.

## Does the paleo diet work?

Studies have shown that the paleo diet works. It is full of healthy, clean, unprocessed food. By cutting out foods such as sugars and carbohydrates, which causes bloat, and processed foods, full of chemicals that should not be put into your body, you are eating the way you should. When eating healthy fats and proteins, you will feel full longer and, therefore, eat less. Also, being plant-based, you will have a great many options of healthy fibers from fruits and vegetables, which will also help you feel satisfied for hours after you eat. The combination of a vegetable-based diet with healthy proteins will help you lose weight, feel full longer, and therefore, lose weight. Plus, with all the healthy vitamins and minerals you get in your diet from eating the right foods, you will have more energy to get through the day. You won't feel the need for energy drinks or extra caffeine. Instead, your diet will provide all that you need.

## How much weight will I lose on the paleo diet?

Weight loss is a very individual process, although

most people who eat on the paleo diet will lose weight. In the first week of the diet, you could lose as much as 5 to 10 pounds, although some of this may be water weight. After the first week, your weight loss should taper off to 1 to 3 pounds per week. Eating the paleo diet regularly will cause your body to naturally shed fat and pounds. Your fat cells will shrink in size. And the best part is that you don't need to cut back calories to do it. Your body will naturally lose fat.

## How long does it take to show results on the paleo diet?

You will start to see weight loss results as soon as the first week on the paleo diet. Although some of this weight loss may be from water weight loss, much of it will also be fat. After the first two weeks, your weight loss will taper to one to two pounds per week.

## What foods are allowed on the paleo diet?

The paleo diet allows certain foods. You are encouraged to eat grass-fed meats, fish and seafood, fresh fruits and vegetables, eggs, nuts and seeds, sweet potatoes and yams, seeds, such as pumpkin or sunflower seeds, and healthful oils. These include olive oils, walnut oils, flaxseed oils, macadamia oil, avocado oil, and coconut oil. In fact, many people substitute coconut or almond milk for dairy milk in their diets, as these items are paleo approved. This diet also allows natural sweeteners such as honey. These are all foods that would have been easily available to humans before the advent of agriculture. They are a normal part of the diet.

# What foods are not allowed on the paleo diet?

Any foods that were not easily available to humans before agriculture are not part of the paleo diet. These foods include grains such as rice, oats, barley, and wheat, beans, legumes, which includes peanuts, dairy products, high-fat processed meats such as hot dogs and bologna, refined sugar products, starchy vegetables such as corn and potatoes, any type of processed foods, processed or refined vegetable oils (such as vegetable or canola oils), and salt. You should also avoid drinking alcohol on the paleo diet.

# Is the paleo diet healthy and safe?

With its emphasis on whole, unprocessed foods, lean meats, plenty of vegetables, and healthy fats, the paleo diet gives you all the nutrients you need to live a healthy life. Your body will thank you for feeding it properly, and you will be rewarded with weight loss, more energy, and a healthier body.

# Chapter 3: Recipes

This section contains some recipes to get you started on the paleo diet. Seven breakfast recipes, seven lunch, seven dinner, and five different desserts are included. As you can see from this selection, the paleo diet allows for a variety of foods to keep your palate happy.

# 7 Breakfast Recipes

**Warrior Omelet**

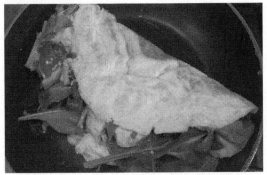

**Serves** 1-2

**Time to prepare:** 10 minutes

**Ingredients:**

- 2 large free range organic eggs, scrambled
- 1 tsp olive oil
- 2 green onions, diced
- 1 cup fresh organic spinach leaves
- 2 organic small tomatoes
- ½ fresh organic avocado sliced into bite sized pieces

**Instructions:**

- Heat olive oil on low in non stick omelet pan.
- Sauté onions until tender.
- Add eggs and cook on low for about 2 minutes.
- Add remaining ingredients.

- Fold and flip omelette until eggs are fully cook

**Nutritional Information:**
Calories: 217, Carbohydrates: 10.5g, Sugar: 3.1g, Fat: 16.9g, Saturated Fat: 3.9g, Protein: 8.4g

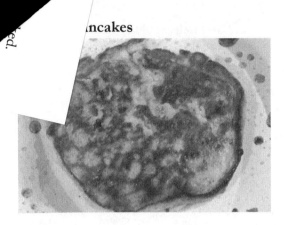

**Serves** 1

**Time to prepare:** 10 minutes

**Ingredients:**

- 1 banana, mashed
- 1 free-range egg
- 1 tsp of coconut, shredded
- 1 tsp cinnamon
- Vanilla Extract, dash (Optional)

**Instructions:**

- Mash one whole banana and lightly beat with an egg.
- For extra flavour, add coconut chips, vanilla extract (just a dash) and cinnamon.
- Pour this mixture into a frying pan and cook as you would a regular pancake.

**Nutritional Information:**
Calories: 187, Carbohydrates: 30.1g, Sugar: 14.6g,
Fat: 5.5g, Saturated Fat: 2.1g, Protein: 7.4g

# Breakfast Scramble

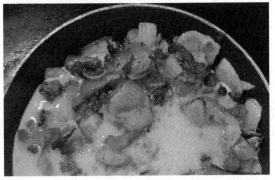

**Serves** 1-2

**Time to prepare:** 20 minutes

## Ingredients:

- 3 Cage-free, non-antibiotic/hormone eggs
- 1/4 – 1/2lb Breakfast sausage, ethically-raised, preservative-free
- 3 Bacon Strips, preservative-free
- 1/2 Onion, diced
- 1/2 – 1 cup Fresh green chilli or salsa (optional if you are avoiding nightshades)

## Instructions:

- Turn on stove top burner to medium heat.
- Layer bacon, sausage bits, and diced onions in a small, non-stick 6-inch frying pan.
- Stir frequently with a wood spatula for 8-12 minutes or until cooked evenly.

- Whisk three eggs in a small mixing bowl.
- Pour egg mixture over bacon, sausage, and onions.
- Stir frequently to avoid burning for 2-4 minutes or until eggs are set.
- Plate egg scramble and garnish with fresh green chilli or salsa

**Nutritional Information:**
Calories: 675, Carbohydrates: 11.2g, Sugar: 5.7g, Fat: 52.5g, Saturated Fat: 16.9g, Protein: 38.6g

## ꞁnd Flour Muffins

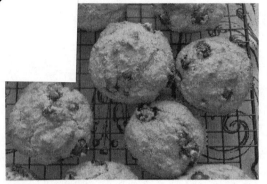

**Serves** 10

**Time to prepare:** 25 minutes

### Ingredients:

- 2-1/2 cups almond flour or almond meal
- ¾ tsp baking soda
- ½ tsp fine sea salt
- 3 large eggs
- ⅓ cup unsweetened pumpkin puree, thawed winter squash puree, butternut squash puree, unsweetened apple sauce, or mashed very ripe banana
- 2 tablespoons honey, agave nectar or maple syrup
- 2 tablespoons coconut oil (melted) or vegetable oil
- 1 teaspoon vinegar (white or cider)
- Optional Flavourings: 1 teaspoon extract (e.g., vanilla, almond), citrus zest, dried herbs (e.g., basil, dill), or spice (e.g., cinnamon, cumin)

- Optional Stir-Ins: 1 cup fresh fruit (e.g., blueberries, diced apple) or ½ cup dried fruit/cacao nibs/chopped nuts/seeds

**Instructions:**

- Preheat oven to 350F. Line 10 cups in a standard 12-cup muffin tin with paper or foil liners.
- In a large bowl whisk the almond flour, baking soda and salt (whisk in any dried spices or herbs at this point, if using).
- In a small bowl, whisk the eggs, pumpkin, honey, oil and vinegar (add any extracts or zest at this point, if using).
- Add the wet ingredients to the dry ingredients, stirring until blended. Fold in any optional stir-ins, if using.
- Divide batter evenly among prepared cups.
- Bake in preheated oven for 14 to 18 minutes until set at the centers and golden brown at the edges. Move the tin to a cooling rack and let muffins cool in the tin 30 minutes. Remove muffins from tin.

**Nutritional Information:**
Calories: 229, Carbohydrates: 10.2g, Sugar: 3.8g, Fat: 17.5g, Saturated Fat: 3g, Protein: 8g

## Paleo Sausage and Sweet Potato Breakfast Casserole

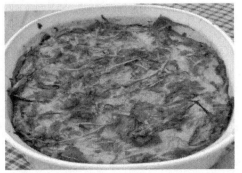

**Serves** 8-10

**Time to prepare:** 70 minutes

### Ingredients

- 1 1/2 lbs. breakfast sausage
- 1/2 tbs coconut oil
- 12 eggs
- 2 sweet potatoes, peeled and diced
- 1/2 large sweet onion, diced
- 1 tsp garlic powder
- 1/4 tsp nutmeg
- 1 tsp. sea salt
- 1 tsp pepper
- 1/4 cup coconut milk
- 4 cups power greens (kale, spinach, arugula)

### Instructions:

- Heat oven to 375 degrees.
- In a large skillet over medium heat, melt coconut oil and add in sausage.
- Brown and break apart with a wooden spoon.
- Beat eggs in extra large bowl.
- Shred sweet potatoes and onion in your food processor. Mix into eggs with seasoning, coconut milk and power greens.
- Grease 9x13 casserole dish with more coconut oil.
- Pour in egg mixture and stir in sausage.
- Cook for 45 minutes. Cover with foil and cook for 10 more minutes or until center is set.

**Nutritional Information:**
Calories: 474, Carbohydrates: 16.2g, Sugar: 1.5g, Fat: 33.4g, Saturated Fat: 12.2g, Protein: 26.8g

# Paleo Yogurt Parfait

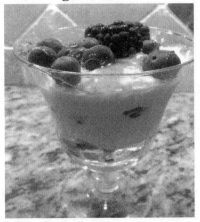

**Serves** 2

**Time to prepare:** 70 minutes

### Ingredients

- 3/4 cup unsalted cashews, soaked in water for 20 minutes
- 1 cup coconut water
- 1 cup meat from inside the coconut
- 1 tsp vanilla.
- Drizzle of honey

### Instructions:

- Start by cracking your coconut and draining the water inside into a small bowl
- Now use a knife to cut out the inner meat of the coconut.

- Pour soaked cashews, coconut water, coconut meat, and vanilla in a blender and mix well
- Serve for breakfast or dessert with blueberries, blackberries, and strawberries. Drizzle honey on top.

**Nutritional Information:**
Calories: 497, Carbohydrates: 36.1g, Sugar: 16.4g, Fat: 37.4g, Saturated Fat: 16.8g, Protein: 10.1g

## Paleo "Oatmeal"

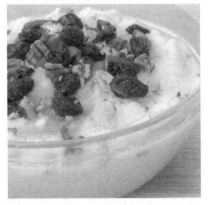

**Serves** 1

**Time to prepare:** 15 minutes

**Ingredients:**

- 1/2 cup full-fat canned coconut milk PLUS 1/4 cup water OR 3/4 cup homemade coconut milk OR 3/4 cup water
- 3 Tbs. coconut flour
- 2 Tbs. finely shredded coconut
- 1 pastured egg OR 1/2 banana, mashed for egg free option
- Oatmeal toppings of your choice

**Instructions:**

- In a small saucepan, mix together the liquid, coconut flour and shredded coconut. Bring to a boil (mixture will be thick), cover, reduce heat to low, and simmer for 2-3 minutes. Stir halfway through.

- Off the heat, crack the egg into the saucepan and whisk quickly to prevent the egg from scrambling with the heat. Then, return to the heat and stir until thickened, about 2 minutes.
- For the egg free version, follow the instructions above but don't add the egg. Instead, whisk in the mashed banana and stir briefly.

**Nutritional Information:**
Calories: 491, Carbohydrates: 21.2g, Sugar: 6.1g, Fat: 40g, Saturated Fat: 33.3g, Protein: 14.1g

# 7 Lunch Recipes

### Chicken salad with balsamic cilantro dressing

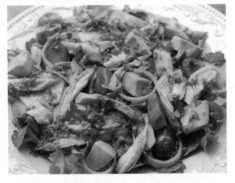

**Serves** 1 person as main entrée salad

**Time to prepare:** 10 minutes

**Ingredients:**

**For the balsamic cilantro dressing:**

- 1-2 tablespoons balsamic vinegar, adjust based on your preference
- 2-3 tablespoons olive oil, adjust based on your preference
- 1 garlic clove, crushed
- 1 tablespoon roughly chopped cilantro
- Salt and pepper to taste

**For the chicken salad:**

- ~2 cups of your choice of mixed salad greens
- ½ avocado, diced or sliced
- 5-6 grape or cherry tomatoes, cut in halves
- A few slices of red onion
- 5-6 slices of cucumber
- ½ cup shredded cooked chicken
- A few coarsely chopped cilantro leaves

**Instructions:**

- To prepare the salad dressing, place the ingredients in a small bowl and whisk lightly. Can be made ahead of time, refrigerate until ready to use.
- To prepare the salad, arrange the mixed salad greens on a large plate, add the diced avocado, tomatoes, red onions, cucumbers, shredded chicken, and the chopped cilantro.
- Pour the balsamic cilantro dressing over the salad, toss and serve immediately.

**Nutritional Information:**
Calories: 625, Carbohydrates: 23.5g, Sugar: 9.4g, Fat: 51g, Saturated Fat: 8g, Protein: 25.3g

# All Meat Veggie Chili

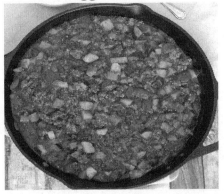

**Serves** 6

**Time to prepare:** 40 minutes

**Ingredients:**

- 1½ pounds grass fed beef (85% is what I use)
- 2 cloves garlic, chopped
- 2 tablespoons oil
- 1 large onion, diced
- 1 stalk celery, chopped
- 4 large carrots, peeled and diced
- 2-3 zucchinis, diced
- 2 tablespoons chilli powder
- 1 teaspoon ground cumin
- 1 teaspoon oregano
- 1 teaspoon salt
- ¼ teaspoon cayenne pepper (optional)
- 15 ounce can tomato puree
- 15 ounce can diced tomatoes

## Instructions:

- In your seasoned skillet or 5-6 quart large cast iron pot, brown beef and garlic. Cook over medium heat until beef is thoroughly cooked and browned. Drain off excess fat, set aside.
- Add oil, onions, celery, carrots, and seasonings to the skillet and cook until translucent over medium high heat, about 5-7 minutes. Once onions are golden and veggies are midway cooked, add zucchinis and cook for 2 minutes making sure you stir everything well.
- Add cooked beef back into the pot, tomatoes, tomato sauce, and stir well. Bring everything to a boil, stirring frequently, reduce heat and simmer for 20 minutes.
- Check on the amazing mixture every so often and stir. Serve immediately.

- **Note**: If you like your chilli with a little more sauce, add another 15 ounce can of tomato sauce.

**Nutritional Information:** Calories: 427, Carbohydrates: 20.8g, Sugar: 10.7g, Fat: 22.6g, Saturated Fat: 7.3g, Protein: 35.2g

# Cucumber and Tomato Salad

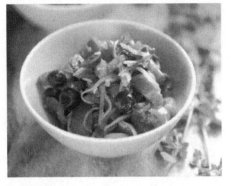

**Serves** 4

**Time to prepare:** 10 minutes

## Ingredients:

- 1 clove Garlic, minced
- 1 cup Kalamata Olives
- 1 Tbsp. fresh Basil, thinly sliced
- 1 Tbsp. fresh Oregano, chopped
- 2 cup Cucumber, cut into noodles with a julienne peeler
- 2 cup Grape Tomatoes
- 2 Tbsp. Balsamic Vinegar
- 2 Tbsp. Extra Virgin Olive Oil
- 1 tsp Black Pepper

## Instructions:

- Rinse and peel cucumber.

- Use julienne peeler to make noodles from the flesh of the cucumber. Stop when you get down to the seeds.
- Rinse grape tomatoes, slice in half.
- Thinly slice basil, chop oregano, and mince garlic.
- Toss all ingredients with the Kalamata olives in a medium mixing bowl, drizzle with olive oil and balsamic vinegar, and sprinkle with black pepper.

**Note**: As an option for this recipe, forgo the olive oil and balsamic vinegar for our balsamic vinaigrette dressing.

### Nutritional Information:
Calories: 130, Carbohydrates: 8.9g, Sugar: 3.3g, Fat: 11g, Saturated Fat: 1.6g, Protein: 1.7g

# Avocado Chicken Salad

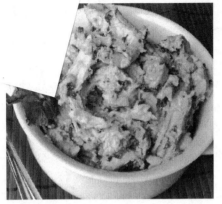

**Serves** 2

**Time to prepare:** 15 minutes

## Ingredients:

- 2 boneless, skinless chicken breasts (cooked and shredded)
- 1/2 cup fresh basil leaves, stems removed
- 2 small or 1 large ripe avocado, pits and skin removed
- 2 Tbsp. extra virgin olive oil
- 1/2 tsp. sea salt (or more to taste)
- 1/8 tsp. ground black pepper (or more to taste)

## Instructions:

- Place the cooked shredded chicken in a medium sized mixing bowl.

- Place the basil, avocado, olive oil, sea salt and ground black pepper in a food processor and blend until smooth. You may need to scrape the sides a couple times to incorporate.
- Pour the avocado and basil mixture into the mixing bowl with the shredded chicken and toss well to coat. Taste and add additional sea salt and ground black pepper if desired. Keep in the fridge until ready to serve.

**Nutritional Information:**
Calories: 632, Carbohydrates: 12.2g, Sugar: 1g, Fat: 45.7g, Saturated Fat: 8.1g, Protein: 45.3g

### Sweet Potato and Kale Chicken Patties

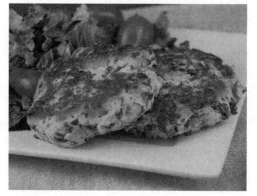

**Serves** 3

**Time to prepare**: 20 minutes (also need 4 hours to allow patties to sit, best prepared the day before)

**Ingredients:**

- 2 green onion, finely chopped
- 1/2 medium sweet potato, peeled and cut into tiny little cubes
- 2 1/2 cups kale, finely chopped (leaves only)
- 1 pound skinless boneless chicken breasts, cut into chunks
- 1/2 teaspoon sea salt
- 1 garlic clove, minced
- 1 teaspoon paprika
- 1 teaspoon Dijon mustard
- 1 tablespoon fresh rosemary, finely chopped
- 1 egg
- 2 tablespoons coconut flour

## Instructions:

- Heat a large skillet over medium high heat with 1 teaspoon coconut oil or avocado oil (or bacon grease) add green onions and cook until tender, about 3 to 5 minutes.
- Add sweet potatoes and cook for 4 to 5 more minutes, until barely tender. Add kale and cook until wilted, about 2 to 3 minutes. Set aside.
- Add chicken to a food processor and process on pulse until ground. Transfer meat to a large mixing bowl. Add salt, garlic, paprika, Dijon mustard, rosemary, egg, coconut flour, and sweet potato mix. Mix together with hands until well combined.
- Cover with plastic wrap and refrigerate for at least 4 hours or even better overnight.
- Divide your chicken mixture into 6 to 7 even patties.
- Coat a large non-stick pan with coconut oil or even better bacon grease to just coat the bottom (not a lot). Add patties and cook until golden crust forms, about 5 to 6 minutes, then flip to the other side and cook until golden and cooked through.

Serve as is or with a side salad.

### Nutritional Information:
Calories: 275, Carbohydrates: 14.8g, Sugar: 2g, Fat: 4.3g, Saturated Fat: 1.2g, Protein: 51.2g

# Chicken Mango Salad

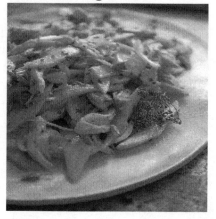

**Serves** 4

**Time to prepare:** 10 minutes

**Ingredients:**

- 8 ounces cooked chicken breast, shredded
- 1 mango, peeled and cut into thin strips
- 1 shallot, julienned
- 2 tablespoons chives
- 2 tablespoons olive oil
- 2 teaspoons honey (or agave)
- 1 lime, zested and juiced
- Kosher salt and pepper

**Instructions:**

- In a medium sized bowl, combine the chives, olive oil, honey and lime juice, whisking together with a fork.
- Add the shredded chicken and the mango and toss together. Season with Salt and pepper to taste and serve chilled.

**Nutritional Information:**
Calories: 207, Carbohydrates: 13.9g, Sugar: 10.9g, Fat: 9.2g, Saturated Fat: 1g, Protein: 18.7g

# Pesto Egg Salad Wraps

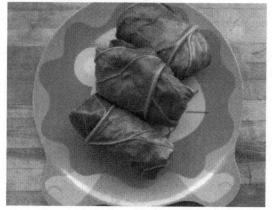

**Serves** 3

**Time to prepare:** 45 minutes

**Ingredients:**

- 3 hardboiled eggs
- 3 large collard leaves
- 1/4 cucumber, diced
- 1/3 c. pesto (recipe below)

**Instructions:**

- Trim the stems off the collard leaves.
- In a large skillet, heat a half inch of water over high heat.
- Add collard leaves and cover. Steam until wilted and "bendy". Remove from water to dry.

- In a bowl, mash together pesto, eggs, and cucumber.
- Place the collard wrap on a clean surface and scoop 1/3 of the egg filling into the center of the leaf. Fold like burrito to make a wrap.
- Do the same with the last 2 leaves.

**Ingredients (**Simple Pesto**):**

- 1 bunch organic basil (cheap at Trader Joe's)
- 3/4- 1 c. extra virgin olive oil
- 1/2 c. walnuts
- Juice of 1/2 lemon
- Sea salt to taste

**Instructions:**

- Put it all in a food processor and blend! Add salt and more lemon juice until reaching the desired taste.

**Nutritional Information:**
Calories: 633, Carbohydrates: 4.4g, Sugar: 1g, Fat: 67.2g, Saturated Fat: 9.3g, Protein: 11.2g

# 7 Dinner Recipes

### Butternut Squash & Kale Beef Stew

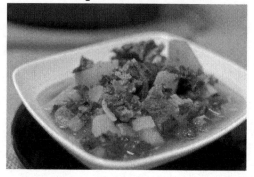

**Serves** 10

**Time to prepare:** 3 hours

**Ingredients:**

- 2 tbsp. bacon fat, or cooking oil of choice
- 2 lb. stew beef, 1" cubed
- 1 onion, roughly chopped
- 4 garlic cloves, minced
- 1 1/2 tbsp. fresh sage, minced
- 1/2 tsp smoked paprika
- 1 small butternut squash, cubed (about 4 cups)
- 16oz frozen, chopped kale (or one bunch fresh)
- 4 cups beef stock, preferably homemade
- Salt and pepper

**Instructions:**

- In a large Dutch oven heat 1 tbsp. bacon fat over medium high. Working in batches, brown the meat, making sure not to cook it through (it can turn tough). Set browned meat aside. Lower heat to medium and add the 2nd tbsp. bacon fat. Once it's melted add the onions, garlic, smoked paprika, and sage to pot, along with a big pinch of salt and fresh pepper. Cook about 8 minutes, or until the onions begin to soften and turn translucent. Make sure to stir frequently so the mixture doesn't burn.
- Add the beef, butternut squash, and kale to the pot. Stir to combine, then add the chicken stock and two cups of hot water. Bring to a boil, then reduce to a simmer and let cook, covered, for at least an hour. I let mine go about 45 minutes longer.

**Nutritional Information:**
Calories: 313, Carbohydrates: 8.4g, Sugar: 0.8g, Fat: 16.3g, Saturated Fat: 3.6g, Protein: 32.2g

# Baked Salmon with Lemon and Thyme

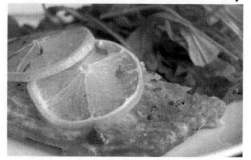

**Serves** 4

**Time to prepare:** 35 minutes

**Ingredients:**

- 32 oz. piece of salmon
- 1 lemon, sliced thin
- 1 tbsp. capers
- Salt and freshly ground pepper
- 1 tbsp. fresh thyme
- Olive oil, for drizzling

**Instructions:**

- Line a rimmed baking sheet with parchment paper and place salmon, skin side down, on the prepared baking sheet. Generously season salmon with salt and pepper. Arrange capers on the salmon, and top with sliced lemon and thyme.

- Place baking sheet in a cold oven, then turn heat to 400 degrees F. Bake for 25 minutes. Serve immediately.

**Nutritional Information:**
Calories: 375, Carbohydrates: 1.9g, Sugar: 0g, Fat: 13.6g, Saturated Fat: 2.2g, Protein: 58.2g

# Grilled Pork Chops with Stone Fruit Slaw

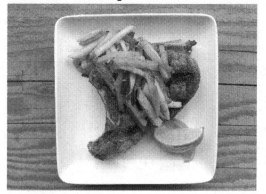

**Serves** 4

**Time to prepare:** 30 minutes

**Ingredients:**

**For the Chops:**

- 4 bone-in pork chops, about 1-1.5 inches thick
- 1 teaspoon sea salt
- 1 teaspoon ground coriander
- 1 teaspoon ground cumin
- 1 teaspoon ground paprika
- For the Slaw:
- 1 pound assorted firm stone fruit (peaches, plums, apricots, etc.)
- 1/4 teaspoon ground chipotle powder (or to taste, this amount will give it a good kick)
- 1 teaspoon lime zest
- 1 teaspoon lime juice

- Pinch sea salt

## Instructions:

- Preheat your grill to medium-high heat and remove your pork chops from the fridge.
- Combine the teaspoon of salt, cumin, coriander and paprika in a small bowl and stir to combine
- Divide the spice rub among the chops, making sure to coat both sides.
- Grill chops for about 5 minutes on each side, or until almost cooked through.
- Alternately, if you don't have a grill, Heat a large skillet over medium-high heat and add your preferred cooking fat (lard would be a good choice here) Sear the chops for 5 minutes on each side, or until almost cooked through.
- Remove to a plate and cover loosely with foil, allowing them to rest for 10 minutes.
- Meanwhile, prepare the slaw: Julienne fruit and place in a medium bowl. Mix in the chipotle powder, lime zest, lime juice, and a pinch of salt. Stir to combine.
- Serve the chops topped with the slaw.

### Nutritional Information:
Calories: 231, Carbohydrates: 12.3g, Sugar: 9.8g, Fat: 9.5g, Saturated Fat: 3g, Protein: 23.2g

# Fennel and Brussels Sprouts Sirloin Rolls

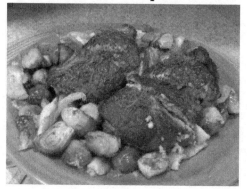

**Serves** 4

**Time to prepare:** 50 minutes

**Ingredients:**

**For the Filling:**

- 2 slices bacon, chopped into 4 or 5 large pieces
- ½ fennel bulb, roughly chopped
- 1/2 cup Brussels sprouts, bottoms trimmed off and halved
- 2 garlic cloves
- 1 tsp each of dried rosemary, sage and oregano

Additional Ingredients:

- 2 ½ lb. sirloin steaks
- Salt and pepper, to taste
- 2 cups Brussels sprouts (about ¾ lb.), bottoms trimmed off and quartered

- ½ fennel bulb, cut into thick slices
- 1 tsp olive oil
- 2 or 3 fennel fronds

**Instructions:**

- Preheat oven to 375F.
- Add all filling ingredients to a food processor. Process until it forms a thick paste.
- Pound out steaks using a mallet until they are about ½ inch thick.
- Spread half of the filling on each steak. Roll steaks up, using a few toothpicks to secure.
- Place sirloin rolls in a large roasting pan and sprinkle with salt and pepper.
- Toss Brussels sprouts and fennel slices in a large bowl with olive oil, salt and pepper.
- Spread Brussels sprouts and fennel slices around sirloin rolls in the roasting pan.
- Roast for 35-40 minutes, until steak is cooked to desired level and vegetables begin to brown. If steak is done and veggies need to cook a bit longer, remove the steak from the pan and let it rest while you cook the veggies for an additional five minutes or so.
- Let steak rest for 5 minutes before slicing. Garnish with fennel fronds.
- 

**Nutritional Information:**
Calories: 641, Carbohydrates: 11.5g, Sugar: 1.6g, Fat: 23.4g, Saturated Fat: 8.2g, Protein: 92.7g

### Paleo Spaghetti Squash & Meatballs

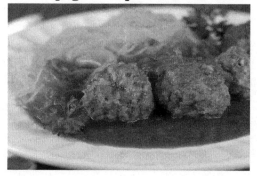

**Serves** 4

**Time to prepare:** 5 hours 30 minutes (5 hours in crock pot)

### Ingredients:

- One medium spaghetti squash.
- One pound of ground Italian sausage.
- One can of tomato sauce, I used a 14 ounce can.
- 2 tbsp. of hot pepper relish (optional).
- 4 to 6 cloves of garlic, whole.
- 2 tbsp. of olive oil.
- Italian seasoning (Oregano, Basil, Thyme) to taste, I used about 2 tsp

### Instructions:

- Make sure you use a large 6 quart slow cooker for this recipe.

- Dump your tomato sauce, olive oil, garlic, hot pepper relish and Italian seasoning into your slow cooker and stir well.
- Cut your squash in half and scoop out the seeds.
- Place your 2 squash halves face down into your slow cooker.
- Roll your ground sausage into meatballs, then fit as many as you can in the sauce around the squash. I was able to work in about a half pound worth.
- Cook on High for 3 hours or cook on low for 5 hours.
- Use a large fork to pull the "spaghetti" out of your squash, then top with your meatballs and sauce.

**Nutritional Information:**
Calories: 473, Carbohydrates: 12.7g, Sugar: 5.1g, Fat: 35.4g, Saturated Fat: 10.2g, Protein: 21.3g

## Paleo Pulled Pork Sliders

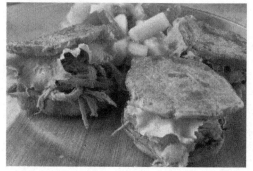

**Serves** 4

**Time to prepare:** 8 hours 30 minutes (8 hours cooking in crock pot)

**Ingredients:**

- Pulled Pork
- Large pork roast
- 1 large onion, sliced
- 3 minced garlic cloves
- 2 tsp cumin
- 2 tsp chilli powder
- 1 tsp pepper
- 2 tsp oregano
- 1 tsp paprika
- 1/2 tsp cayenne pepper
- 1/2 tsp cinnamon
- 2 tsp sea salt
- Juice of 1 lime
- Juice of 1 lemon

## Instructions:

- Stir together the spices and rub all over the roast. Lay the onion slices down on the bottom of the slow cooker, and squeeze half of the fruit juices in. Put the roast in the crockpot and squeeze the remaining lime and lemon juice over it. Cook on low overnight or throughout the day about 8 hours (you really can't overcook it to be honest). When done, shred it with two forks until it's completely 'pulled'.

## Ingredients:

- The "Buns"
- 1 large sweet potato (try to go for a nice evenly round one, remember the diameter will be the size of your sliders)
- 2 tbsp. coconut oil
- 1/4 tsp cumin
- 1/4 tsp paprika
- Dash of sea salt

## Instructions:

- Slice the sweet potato into 1/4″ thick rounds. Lay them out on a parchment paper-lined cookie sheet.
- Brush each slice with coconut oil and sprinkle with the spices, then flip and do the same on the other side.
- Bake at 425 degrees Fahrenheit for 35 minutes until golden brown on the outside and cooked all

the way through, flipping halfway through. You may need to crank it up to 450.

- Top a patty with pulled pork, and add any other toppings or sauces you'd
- Finish with the top patty and enjoy.

**Nutritional Information:**

Calories: 220, Carbohydrates: 16.2g, Sugar: 4.8g, Fat: 11.6g, Saturated Fat: 7.4g, Protein: 14.2g

# Paleo Crockpot Jambalaya Soup

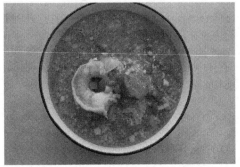

**Serves** 6

**Time to prepare:** 6 hours 30 minutes (6 hours in crock pot)

## Ingredients:

- 5 cups chicken stock.
- 4 peppers – any color you want, chopped
- 1 large onion, chopped
- 1 large can of organic diced tomatoes (leave the juice)
- 2 cloves garlic, diced
- 2 bay leafs
- 1 lb. large shrimp, raw and de-veined.
- 4 oz. chicken, diced
- 1 package spicy Andouille sausage
- 1/2-1 head of cauliflower
- 2 c. okra (optional)
- 3 tbsp. Cajun Seasoning

- 1/4 c. Frank's Red Hot (or hot sauce of your choice)

**Instructions:**

- Put the chopped peppers, onions, garlic, chicken, Cajun seasoning, Red Hot, and bay leafs in the crockpot with the chicken stock. As you can see, I grabbed a container of my homemade stock directly from the freezer and threw it in. Set on low for 6 hours.
- About 30 minutes before it's finished, toss in the cut up sausages.
- While this is cooking quickly make cauliflower rice by pulsing raw cauliflower in the food processor until it resembles rice.
- For the last 20 minutes, add in the cauliflower rice and the raw shrimp. Note: You can choose to quickly steam the cauliflower rice in the microwave and serve the jambalaya OVER it as well.

**Nutritional Information:**
Calories: 307, Carbohydrates: 12.6g, Sugar: 5.2g, Fat: 16.4g, Saturated Fat: 3.3g, Protein: 29.2g

# 5 Dessert Recipes

## Baked Cinnamon Apple Chips

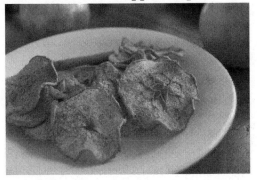

**Serves** 2

**Time to prepare:** 3 hours

**Ingredients:**

- 2 apples (I used Honey crisp)
- 1 tsp cinnamon

**Instructions:**

- Preheat oven to 200 degrees.
- Using a sharp knife or mandolin, slice apples thinly. Discard seeds. Prepare a baking sheet with parchment paper and arrange apple slices on it without overlapping. Sprinkle cinnamon over apples.

- Bake for approximately 1 hour, then flip. Continue baking for 1-2 hours, flipping occasionally, until the apple slices are no longer moist. Store in airtight container.

**Nutritional Information**:
Calories: 113, Carbohydrates: 30.2g, Sugar: 22.1g, Fat: 0.4g, Saturated Fat: 0g, Protein: 0.6g

# Chocolate Mug Cake

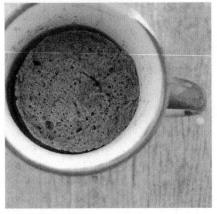

**Serves** 1

**Time to prepare:** 3 minutes

**Ingredients:**

* 1 heaping tbsp. almond flour
* 1 heaping tbsp. unsweetened cocoa powder
* 1 tbsp. almond milk (I used unsweetened vanilla)
* ½ tbsp. honey
* 1 egg
* 1 tsp vanilla extract

**Instructions:**

* It really is so delightfully simple! Mix all ingredients together in a mug and microwave for 1-1.5 minutes.

- Serve with your favorite nut butter or ice cream and enjoy!

**Nutritional Information:**
Calories: 314, Carbohydrates: 19.3g, Sugar: 11.1g, Fat: 22.7g, Saturated Fat: 6g, Protein: 13g

# Raw Brownie Bites

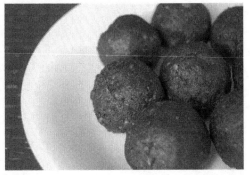

**Serves** 10

**Time to prepare:** 10 minutes

## Ingredients:

- 1 1/2 cups walnuts
- Pinch of salt
- 1 cup pitted dates
- 1 tsp vanilla
- 1/3 cup unsweetened cocoa powder

## Instructions:

- Add walnuts and salt to a blender or food processor. Mix until the walnuts are finely ground.
- Add the dates, vanilla, and cocoa powder to the blender. Mix well until everything is combined. With the blender still running, add a couple drops of water at a time to make the mixture stick together.

- Using a spatula, transfer the mixture into a bowl. Using your hands, form small round balls, rolling in your palm. Store in an airtight container in the refrigerator for up to a week.

**Nutritional Information:**
Calories: 174, Carbohydrates: 16.8g, Sugar: 11.6g, Fat: 11.5g, Saturated Fat: 0.9g, Protein: 5.5g

# Grilled Peaches with Coconut Cream

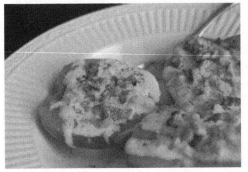

**Serves** 6

**Time to prepare:** 15 minutes

**Ingredients:**

- 3 medium ripe peaches, cut in half with pit removed
- 1 tsp vanilla
- 1 can coconut milk, refrigerated
- 1/4 cup chopped walnuts
- Cinnamon (to taste)

**Instructions:**

- Place peaches on the grill with the cut side down first. Grill on medium-low heat until soft, about 3-5 minutes on each side.
- Scoop cream off the top of the can of chilled coconut milk. Whip together coconut cream and vanilla with handheld mixer. Drizzle over each

peach. Top with cinnamon and chopped walnuts to garnish.

**Nutritional Information:**
Calories: 145, Carbohydrates: 7.5g, Sugar: 5.6g, Fat: 12.7g, Saturated Fat: 8.7g, Protein: 2.6g

# Almond Joy Ice Cream

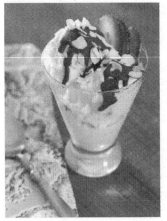

**Serves** 6

**Time to prepare:** 25 minutes (needs to chill overnight)

**Ingredients:**

- 2 cans full fat coconut milk
- ½ cup honey
- 1 ½ tablespoons vanilla extract
- 1 dark baking chocolate bar
- ¼ cup sliced almonds
- ½ cup unsweetened coconut flakes

**Instructions:**

- In a blender, mix together the coconut milk, honey, and vanilla extract. Line a plastic Tupperware with plastic wrap. Pour the mixture into it and freeze it overnight. The next day, take half of the frozen mixture and add it to a food processor. Mix it on high until it resembles frozen yogurt and put it back into a storage container. Repeat this process with the other half of the mixture. Return the blended ice cream to the freeze for 30 minutes before serving.

- To assemble, melt the chocolate chips in a saucepan over low heat, to prevent burning the chocolate. Serve each Almond Joy Sunday with a scoop of the ice cream. Drizzle the melted chocolate on top, then sprinkle with coconut flakes and sliced almonds. Serve immediately.

**Nutritional Information:**
Calories: 218, Carbohydrates: 27.2g, Sugar: 24.8g, Fat: 11.3g, Saturated Fat: 8.5g, Protein: 1.9g

# Conclusion:

Delicious recipes that nourish the body and soul. Foods that are clean, pure, and perfect for staying in shape. Recipes that encourage weight loss, fill you up for hours at a time, and make you feel better and more energetic. These are all positive aspects of the paleo diet. By eating healthy, unprocessed foods, the way they were intended, you will lose weight, feel healthier, and have more energy. It is one of the healthiest ways to eat. Simply following the paleo plan, eating only when you are hungry, and assuring that your foods contain lean meats, healthy fats, and a great variety of vegetables, you will lose weight and feel better. Take control of your life! The paleo diet will lead you to a healthier, happier life.

Thanks again for reading. Here's to a healthier you!<u>Don't forget to grab our free weight loss report to maximize your chances of success!</u>

Finally, if you enjoyed this book, then I'd like to ask you for a favor: would you be kind enough to leave a review for this book on Amazon? It'd be greatly appreciated!

<u>Click here to leave a review for this book on Amazon!</u>
Thank you and good luck!

# You may also like these books...

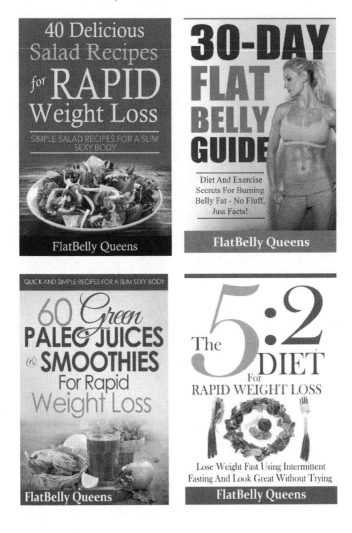

Made in the USA
San Bernardino, CA
24 September 2017